Jessica F. Turner

Dental Care Revolution

Natural Whitening and Cleaning Procedures

tredition

Disclaimer:

This content is not intended to be taken as medical advice or a suggestion for a course of treatment; rather, it is presented solely for informational purposes. It is not intended to serve as a replacement for the diagnosis or treatment provided by a trained medical professional or dentist.

Both the author of this material and the publisher of it disclaim any responsibility for individual choices or actions taken in reliance on the information that is provided. In the event of any health complaints or concerns, one should never hesitate to speak with a qualified medical or dental professional.

Before making any adjustments to one's health or course of treatment, it is strongly advised that one confer with a trained medical professional regarding any and all information and recommendations. There will be no responsibility taken for any injuries or damages that may occur as a direct or indirect result of using the information that has been provided.

Contents

Foreword

Dear Readers,

I am Jessica F. Turner. In my role as author of this book, I would like to take this opportunity to introduce myself to you not only as an authority in the field of natural dental care but also as a patient who has endured its effects. For a significant amount of time, I struggled with a wide variety of dental issues. My teeth and gums were hypersensitive to the majority of dental care products that are available for purchase, which was another thing that caused me a lot of pain and discomfort. Some of you are probably familiar with the unpleasant side effects such as burning, itching, and irritation.

Instead of experiencing relief, I frequently felt powerless and like I was caught in a never-ending cycle. I wished to take better care of and protect my teeth, but I kept running into obstacles. It seemed as though I had no choice but to make a decision between having healthy teeth and having an oral cavity free of symptoms.

My own personal journey has finally caused me to question the traditional approach that is taken to dental care. I started looking for other options, as well as intensively researching and experimenting with different natural care techniques. What started out as a quest for personal relief quickly turned into a deep passion for discovering how the gifts of nature can help us maintain and improve our oral health.

In this book, I share with you my findings, experiences, and the wonderful alternatives to conventional dental care that are not only gentle and tolerable, but are also effective. These alternatives are not only effective, but they are also tolerable. My intention is to give you a comprehensive handbook that will serve as a guide as you make your way toward oral care that is less artificial and more natural.

I am grateful for your trust, and I hope that you have an enlightening read and teeth that are sparklingly healthy.

yours,

Jessica F. Turner

1. Introduction to dental health and natural care.

Dental health is much more than just a bright smile or the absence of toothache. A healthy set of teeth plays a central role in our overall well-being and impacts many aspects of our lives - from the way we eat to the quality of our communication with others.

Nutrient absorption and digestion

Our teeth are the first link in the food chain. They break down food into smaller pieces that can then be digested more easily. If our teeth are not functioning properly - whether through disease, misalignment or loss - it can affect the way we eat and therefore the type of nutrients we absorb. Healthy dental health ensures efficient food intake and optimal digestion.

Self-awareness and social interactions

A healthy set of teeth also influences our self-image and self-confidence. People who are proud of their smile tend to smile more, which in turn promotes positive social interactions. In contrast, problems with the teeth - such as discoloration, missing teeth or bad breath - can affect self-confidence and prevent us from fully engaging in social situations.

Link to general health

There is also growing evidence that dental health is closely linked to overall health. For example, inflammation in the mouth, as occurs with periodontitis, can lead to systemic inflammation throughout the body, which in turn has been linked to a variety of diseases, including heart disease and diabetes.

In a fictional case study called "Anna's Experience," Anna, a 45-year-old teacher, experienced recurrent sore throats and difficulty swallowing. A visit to an otolaryngologist revealed that the cause of her discomfort was not in her throat, but in her mouth. Advanced periodontitis had affected not only her gums but also other parts of her body.

Prevention is better than cure

The key to maintaining dental health is prevention. Regular dental checkups, good oral hygiene at home and a balanced diet are crucial to preventing dental problems before they even start.

In summary, dental health should not be viewed in isolation. It is a reflection of our overall health and well-being. A healthy set of teeth not only contributes to a beautiful smile, but also to a healthy life. By caring for and protecting our teeth, we are actually doing much more: investing in our overall health and quality of life.

Relationship between dental health and general health

The oral cavity is not only the place where digestion begins; it is also a window into our overall health. The importance of dental health goes far beyond an attractive smile; it can actually provide clues to the state of our entire body and even increase certain disease risks.

A mirror of the body condition

Dentists can sometimes detect the first signs of disease. For example, paler gums or excessive bleeding from the gums can be signs of blood disorders or even anemia. Similarly, dry mouth may indicate diabetes or other hormonal disorders.

The role of bacteria

Our mouth is home to millions of bacteria, most of which are harmless. However, if oral hygiene is poor, harmful bacteria can multiply and lead to gum disease. These bacteria can then enter the bloodstream and cause inflammation and infection in other parts of the body.

Cardiovascular diseases

There is evidence that inflammatory diseases of the mouth, such as periodontitis, are associated with an increased risk of heart disease. It is suspected that inflammation in the mouth can lead to inflammation in the blood vessels, which in turn increases the risk of cardiovascular disease.

Consider, for example, the fictional story of Marco, a 50-year-old man. Marco had periodontitis for years and thought it was a purely dental problem. Years later, he was diagnosed with heart disease. While it is hard to say whether there was a direct link between his dental disease and his heart disease, research shows that there are possible links.

Pregnancy and birth

Gum disease can increase the risk of premature birth or low birth weight. It is believed that the inflammation and infection in the mouth can affect the uterus, which could lead to such complications.

Osteoporosis

Osteoporosis, a disease that causes brittle and porous bones, may also be associated with tooth loss and periodontitis, as the jawbone may also be affected by the disease.

Endocarditis

This is an infection of the inner lining of the heart. It usually occurs when bacteria or other germs from another part of the body, such as the mouth, enter the heart through the bloodstream.

In conclusion, our dental health can have far-reaching effects on our overall health. Not only is it important to visit the dentist regularly, but also to consider oral health as an integral part of our overall well-being. A healthy mouth can pave the way to a healthier body.

How conventional dental care works and where it fails

Conventional dental care, as practiced by many people around the world, has evolved and refined over the years to meet various needs and requirements. It is based on an interplay of daily routine at home and regular professional dental visits. However, despite its widespread acceptance and successes, there are also aspects in which the conventional method shows weaknesses.

The mechanics of conventional dental care

The basic principle of conventional dental care includes mechanical cleaning of the teeth. This means that brushing and flossing remove plaque and food debris. Toothpastes containing fluoride help to strengthen tooth enamel and prevent caries. Dental check-ups allow problems to be detected and treated at an early stage.

Strengths of the conventional method

- Prophylaxis: Conventional dental care has proven to be extremely effective in preventing caries and gum disease.
- Scientifically sound: Many products recommended for conventional dental care are the result of decades of research and testing.
- Wide availability: Conventional care products are available almost everywhere, which facilitates their use.

Weak points of conventional dental care

- Chemicals and additives: Many dental care products contain a number of chemicals, including preservatives, artificial sweeteners and colorants, which some people may want to avoid.
- Overemphasis on mechanics: While mechanical brushing is important, brushing too aggressively can damage gums or cause them to recede.
- Environmental impact: The production and disposal of toothbrushes, dental floss and toothpaste tubes has an ecological impact, particularly with regard to plastic waste.

For example, consider the fictional case study of Lara, an environmentally conscious mother of two. Lara noticed that despite her consistent dental care and buying the "best" branded products, her children kept developing cavities. After some research, she came across information about certain additives in conventional

Toothpastes that could influence the pH value in the mouth.

Conclusion

Conventional dental care undoubtedly offers numerous benefits and has protected and improved the smiles of many people. But as with many things, there is room for improvement and alternatives. In an age where awareness of health and the environment is growing, more and more people are looking for ways to adapt their dental care to their individual needs and beliefs.

Definition and principles of natural dental care

Natural dental care takes a holistic approach that includes not only mechanical cleaning, but also the use of natural, often biodegradable products and the promotion of a healthy oral environment through diet and lifestyle habits.

Definition

Natural dental care is the approach of maintaining and promoting the health of teeth and gums through natural methods and means. This excludes the use of chemical additives and artificial substances and relies on ingredients that come from nature.

The basic principles of natural dental care

1. Prevention: Before problems even arise, supporters of natural dental care focus on prevention. This can be supported by a balanced diet rich in minerals and vitamins.

2. Use of natural products: Instead of fluoride toothpastes or mouthwashes with alcohol, advocates rely on alternatives such as coconut oil, baking soda or herbal extracts.
3. Mechanical cleaning: Even when natural dental care products are used, mechanical cleaning through brushing and flossing remains a key aspect. However, there are also sustainable alternatives to conventional plastic toothbrushes, such as bamboo toothbrushes.
4. Preservation of the natural oral environment: The mouth is an ecosystem. Natural dental care strives to maintain this balance instead of disturbing it with aggressive products.
5. Connection of body and mind: For many followers of natural dental care, emotional and mental health also play a role. Stress, for example, can lead to teeth grinding at night, so relaxation techniques can be an integral part of this approach.
6. Environmental awareness: Many who choose natural dental care also do so out of an ecological awareness. They choose products that have been produced sustainably and generate little or no plastic waste.

A practical example: Let's take the imaginary story of Lea. Lea, who lives in a rural community, has always been interested in the environment and her own health. Instead of using commercial toothpaste, she uses a mixture of coconut oil and turmeric. She has found that this mixture not only cleans her teeth, but also leaves a pleasant feeling in her mouth. In addition, Lea uses a bamboo toothbrush and relies on homemade mouthwashes made from herbal teas.

Final thoughts

Natural dental care goes beyond simply brushing the teeth. It views the mouth as a part of the entire body and emphasizes holistic health and sustainability. This approach can not only lead to better oral health, but also help to raise awareness of one's own body and the environment.dental care to their individual needs and beliefs.

Why you should consider natural dental care

At a time when our lives are dominated by technology and synthetic products, many long for a return to nature, to the simple and genuine. This longing extends not only to our diet or cosmetics, but also to our dental care. But why swap out the conventional remedies on your bathroom countertop for natural alternatives in the first place? Here are some reasons to switch to natural dental care.

- Avoidance of chemicals and additives: Many conventional dental care products contain ingredients whose names are difficult to pronounce and whose effects and side effects are often unclear. Natural products, on the other hand, rely on simple, easy-to-understand ingredients.

- Protection of the oral ecosystem: Our oral cavity is a sensitive ecosystem. Overly aggressive or artificial substances can disturb this balance. Natural products are often gentler and support the natural environment.
- Sustainability and environmental protection: Natural dental care products are often packaged in a more environmentally friendly way and leave less waste. In addition, they are usually produced without animal testing.
- Holistic approach: Natural dental care does not consider the mouth in isolation, but in the context of the entire body. This can contribute to a better overall well-being.
- Personalization: Natural dental care leaves room for individuality. Whether you prefer coconut oil, baking soda or a mixture of both - you can adapt your care to your own needs.
- Economic considerations: Although some natural products may be more expensive to purchase, they can save you money in the long run by reducing the number of products you need and reducing potential dental treatments due to better preventive care.

A thought experiment: Imagine Erik, a man in his mid-forties who repeatedly struggled with gum problems. After trying several conventional products, he decided to try a natural method: a rinse made from diluted tea tree oil. After a few weeks, he noticed that his gum problems subsided significantly and he generally felt better.

Summary

Choosing natural dental care is not just a trend, but is based on concrete benefits for both individual health and the environment. It's a conscious choice that can pave the way for a more sustainable and healthier life. If you're looking for ways to make your life more conscious and natural, switching to natural dental care could be an excellent first step.

Advantages of natural dental care

Choosing to rethink the way we care for our teeth can have far-reaching benefits. Especially when you leave the traditional path and turn to natural dental care. But what exactly makes this approach so special?

- Less toxicity: Natural dental care products often contain fewer or no synthetic preservatives, dyes or other additives that could potentially be toxic. This means less exposure to potentially harmful chemicals.
-
- Gentle on sensitive mouths: Without harsh chemicals or alcohols, natural products are often gentler on people with sensitive gums or teeth.
- Environmentally friendly: Natural dental care often relies on environmentally friendly packaging and ingredients that are biodegradable. This reduces the ecological footprint and promotes a sustainable lifestyle.

- Fewer allergic reactions: Because natural dental care products contain fewer synthetic ingredients, allergic reactions or intolerances are less common.
- Supports microbiome health: The mouth has its own microbiome - a community of microorganisms that live in a delicate balance. Natural dental care supports this balance rather than upsetting it.
- Avoidance of antibiotic resistance: Some oral care products contain antimicrobials that can contribute to the development of antibiotic-resistant bacteria. Natural alternatives often circumvent this risk.
- Holistic benefits: Incorporating natural dental care into daily life often makes people aware of other health- and environmentally-conscious habits, which can lead to a more holistic approach to wellness.
- Cost-efficiency: Although first impressions sometimes suggest otherwise, natural products can save money in the long run. They are often more concentrated and versatile and can be used for multiple applications.

Imagine the fictional Sarah, a young mother who decided to rethink her lifestyle. She chose natural dental care products, not only for herself, but also for her children. Over time, she noticed that not only did her family's teeth appear brighter, but their gums were healthier as well. Her children had fewer toothaches, and she herself felt reassured knowing that she wasn't exposing her family to unnecessary chemicals.

Conclusion

Natural dental care offers a wealth of benefits that consider both health and the environment. By choosing natural alternatives, you're making a statement for yourself, your family and the planet. It's a small step with a big impact. A step towards a more conscious and healthier life.

2. Understanding of the mouth and its functions

Our oral cavity is much more than just the place where our meals begin. It is a complex system of bones, muscles, salivary glands and, of course, teeth, all working together harmoniously to perform a variety of tasks. Let's dive into the fascinating anatomy of the mouth and its components.

- The mouth (oral cavity): Before we turn to the teeth, let's start with the general structure of the mouth. The oral cavity extends from the lips to the beginning of the throat and from one cheek to the other.
- The gums (gingiva): The gums are the soft tissues that surround the teeth and hold them in place. Healthy gums are firm, pink and do not bleed when brushing or eating.
- Teeth: People have two sets of teeth during their lifetime - milk teeth and permanent teeth. There are different types of teeth, each with specific functions:
  - Incisors (incisivi): Located in front, used for cutting food.
  - Canine teeth (kanini): These more pointed teeth tear food.
  - Premolar teeth (premolars): These grind and grind food.
  - Grinding teeth (molars): The largest teeth, mainly for grinding food.

- The tongue: A muscular organ that helps with chewing, swallowing and speaking. It also contains thousands of taste buds that allow us to detect different flavors.
- The palate: Divided into the hard palate at the front and the soft palate at the back. The hard palate separates the oral cavity from the nasal cavity, while the soft palate helps with swallowing.
- Salivary glands: There are three main pairs of salivary glands - the parotid, submandibular and sublingual glands. Saliva contains enzymes that help in the digestive process and keep the mouth moist.
- The temporomandibular joint (TMG): This joint connects the lower jaw to the temporal bone of the skull and allows us to open and close the mouth.

A small example: Think of Thomas eating a crusty baguette. When he bites down, his incisors use their sharp edges to cut through the bread. Then, as he chews, the premolars and molars take over the task of crushing the bread. At the same time, the tongue mixes the bread with saliva to start the digestive process and make swallowing easier.

Conclusion

The anatomy of our mouth is both complex and impressive. Each part has a specific and important function that allows us to eat, speak and breathe. By better understanding these structures, we can better appreciate the importance of oral care and place more value on our daily oral hygiene.

Physiological processes in the mouth: salivation, digestion and more

The mouth is much more than just the entrance to our digestive system. In this small area of our body, numerous physiological processes take place that are essential for our health and well-being.

Salivation:

What is saliva? Saliva is a clear liquid that consists mainly of water, but also contains enzymes, electrolytes, mucus and antibacterial compounds.

Function: It plays a key role in digestion by softening foods and providing the enzyme amylase, which initiates the breakdown of carbohydrates. Saliva also helps balance the pH in the mouth, remineralize teeth and fight pathogens.

Pre-digestion:

As soon as we eat, the digestion process actually begins in our mouth. The mechanical comminution of food by chewing combined with the enzymatic activity of saliva ensures that the food is broken down into smaller, more easily digestible particles.

Taste:

Our tongue is equipped with thousands of taste buds that enable us to detect flavors such as sweet, sour, bitter, salty and umami. These taste buds send signals to the brain that tell us not only the taste, but also the texture and temperature of the food.

Antibacterial activity:

Our mouth is constantly exposed to pathogens. Fortunately, saliva has antibacterial properties, which are supported by enzymes such as lysozyme and immunological proteins such as immunoglobulins. These help keep the growth of harmful microbes in check.

Thermoregulation:

The mouth also helps regulate body temperature. During physical exertion or high temperatures, panting or sucking ice can help cool the body.

A small example: Take Anna, who is biting into a piece of juicy watermelon. Immediately, her saliva starts flowing, softening the flesh and beginning to break down the carbohydrates contained in the watermelon. The taste buds on her tongue send a signal to her brain that what she is eating is sweet and refreshing. And while she enjoys, the antibacterial components of her saliva fight any harmful microorganisms that may be present.

Conclusion

The oral cavity is a place of wonder. The various physiological processes that take place here are both fascinating and essential to our overall health. A deeper understanding of these processes can inspire us to take even better care of our oral health.

How diet and lifestyle influence dental health

Our mouth is the gateway to our body and often reflects the state of our overall health. While daily dental care is crucial, our diet and lifestyle habits also play a supporting role in the health of our gums and teeth.

1. Nutrition: a double sword

- Sugar and carbohydrates: These are the main food for the bacteria in our mouth. When they break down sugar, they produce acids that can erode tooth enamel. This can lead to tooth decay.
- Calcium-rich foods: Milk, cheese and yogurt are not only good for the bones. They also help strengthen tooth enamel and prevent tooth decay.
- Vitamin C: This vitamin, abundant in citrus fruits, peppers and broccoli, strengthens gums and helps prevent gum disease.
- Crunchy foods: apples, carrots and celery act like a natural toothbrush and help remove plaque from teeth.

2. Hydration

- Water: Drinking water, especially after meals, can help flush harmful acids and food debris that would otherwise remain between teeth.
- Reduce acidic drinks: soft drinks, juices and even some teas can erode teeth. It is wise to consume them in moderation and rinse your mouth with water afterwards.

3. Lifestyle and habits

- Smoking: Tobacco use is one of the main enemies of gums. It increases the risk of gum disease and can lead to tooth loss.

- Alcohol: Excessive alcohol consumption can dry out the mouth, increasing the risk of tooth decay and gum disease.
- Mouthguards: For people who play contact sports, a mouthguard can significantly reduce the risk of dental injury.
- Regular dental check-ups: Despite good nutrition and lifestyle habits, regular check-ups are essential to detect potential problems early.

A concise example: Consider Tom, an avid runner who eats a balanced diet but has a weakness for energy drinks. Although he brushes his teeth regularly, he notices increased sensitivity in his teeth. A visit to the dentist reveals incipient erosion damage from the acids in his drinks. Tom decides to reduce his consumption and drink water after each energy drink to neutralize the acids.

Common oral and dental problems and their causes

The health of our mouth is a reflection of our overall health and lifestyle habits. A variety of problems can develop in the mouth and teeth, many of which can be prevented with regular preventive care and proper oral hygiene. Here are some of the most common problems and their causes:

1. caries

Causes: Dental caries, often referred to as "tooth decay," occurs when teeth are eroded by acids produced by oral bacteria. These acids are formed when bacteria break down sugars and starches from food.

2. gum disease

Causes: They are caused by an accumulation of plaque at the gumline. If this plaque is not removed, it can cause gingivitis, which can lead to more serious conditions such as periodontitis.

3. oral thrush

Causes: A fungus called Candida albicans causes this infection. It often occurs in people with weakened immune systems or in infants.

4. dry mouth

Causes: Decreased saliva production can be caused by medications, certain diseases or radiation therapy. Saliva is essential to keep the mouth moist and to ward off bacteria.

5. tooth erosion

Causes: Consumption of acidic foods and beverages, such as citrus fruits and soft drinks, can erode tooth enamel.

6. sensitive teeth

Causes: This can be caused by eroded enamel, gum recession, or an aggressive tooth brushing technique.

7. bad breath (halitosis)

Causes: While there are many causes, some of the most common are: poor oral hygiene, dry mouth, gum disease, or eating certain foods like garlic or onions.

8. tooth discoloration

Causes: Some of the main culprits are tobacco, coffee, tea and red wine. But poor oral care can also lead to discoloration.

To illustrate: Consider Anna, a 28-year-old marketing professional. Anna loves her morning coffee and often drinks lemonade with lunch. She notices that her teeth are becoming more sensitive and taking on a yellowish tinge. During a visit to the dentist, she learns that the combination of acid from the lemonade and the discoloration from the coffee is causing these problems.

The link between oral health and diseases such as diabetes and heart disease

Our oral health is closely linked to the overall well-being of our body. What happens in the mouth does not always stay there. Diseases and conditions in the mouth can impact the entire body, and conversely, systemic diseases can impact the condition of our mouth. Two such diseases that interact remarkably with oral health are diabetes and heart disease.

1. diabetes and oral health

Diabetes is a chronic disease that affects the body's sugar metabolism. People with diabetes are at increased risk for various health problems, and these include mouth-related complications.

- Gum disease: People with diabetes are more susceptible to gingivitis and periodontitis. Elevated blood glucose levels can reduce the body's ability to fight infections, making the gums more susceptible to infection.

- Dry mouth: Another common problem in diabetics is dry mouth caused by decreased saliva flow. This can lead to increased plaque formation, gum disease and oral thrush.
- Delayed healing: People with diabetes heal more slowly, which can lead to complications after dental procedures.

2. heart disease and oral health

- Heart disease is a group of conditions that affect the heart and blood vessels. Surprisingly, studies indicate that there is a link between gum disease and heart disease.
- Inflammation: Research has shown that gingivitis can lead to systemic inflammation in the body, which in turn increases the risk of heart disease.
- Bacteria: Bacteria from inflamed gums can enter the bloodstream and build up in the arteries of the heart, leading to atherosclerosis (hardening of the arteries).

For example, imagine Lukas, a 52-year-old businessman. Lukas has had uncontrolled diabetes for years and also neglects his oral care. Recently, he was diagnosed with heart disease. His doctor stressed the importance of good oral care, explaining that an unhealthy oral cavity can affect heart health.

The journey into the deep connection between oral health and systemic diseases such as diabetes and heart disease continues. In the previous section, we looked at the impact of diabetes on oral health and the link between gum disease and heart disease. Here, we will dive deeper and look at other aspects of this complex interaction.

1. oral health as an early indicator

Oral problems can often serve as early warning signs of systemic diseases. For example, inflamed gums and sores in the mouth that are slow to heal may indicate diabetes. Similarly, people with chronic periodontitis, a severe form of gum disease, may be at higher risk for cardiovascular disease.

2. complications due to common risk factors.

Smoking, an unbalanced diet and lack of physical activity are risk factors that can affect both oral health and general health. Smoking, for example, significantly increases the risk of gum disease and heart disease.

3. drug interactions

Some medications used to treat heart disease, such as calcium channel blockers, can cause side effects such as gum enlargement. Diabetics taking insulin or other medications may also notice changes in their mouth.

A real life case (fictional)

Consider Anna, a 45-year-old teacher. Anna began noticing regular bleeding and swelling of her gums. During her dental visit, she was told about the risk of gum disease due to her type 2 diabetes. After further testing, her primary care physician determined that she was also susceptible to cardiovascular disease. This example shows how closely oral health and general health are linked and how one can influence the other.

Protection and prevention

To minimize the risk of both oral and systemic diseases, it is essential:

- Maintain good oral hygiene
- Perform regular dental checkups
- Avoid risk factors such as smoking and poor dietary habits
- Seek proper medical care for pre-existing conditions such as diabetes

3. Natural teeth cleaning

While many of us consider daily tooth cleaning a chore, it is actually a fundamental aspect of our overall health care. The importance of conscientious oral care extends far beyond the mere pursuit of a dazzling smile.

1. the fight against bacteria

Our oral cavity is a vibrant ecosystem full of microorganisms. Without regular cleaning, harmful bacteria can accumulate and lead to plaque, a sticky substance that attaches itself to the teeth. Not only does plaque look unsightly - it is also the main cause of tooth decay.

2. prevention of gum disease

Gum disease, such as gingivitis, results from inflamed gums due to bacterial buildup. If not treated, it can lead to more serious conditions such as periodontitis, which can affect the structures that support the tooth.

3. fresh breath

No one wants to have bad breath. Regular brushing and flossing help remove food debris and bacteria that can cause bad odor.

4. preservation of the natural whiteness of the teeth

Over time, stains can form on the teeth due to coffee, tea, red wine and other foods. Thorough cleaning helps to minimize such discoloration and preserve the natural whiteness of the teeth.

Example of a fictitious patient: Moritz

Moritz, an avid coffee drinker, noticed yellowish discoloration on his teeth one day. Although he brushed twice a day, he neglected to floss. After he realized the importance of thoroughly cleaning his teeth and incorporated flossing into his routine, not only did the color of his teeth improve, but his gums became healthier as well.

5. prevention of major health problems.

Poor oral hygiene can also lead to more serious health problems. There is a known link between oral health and heart disease, diabetes and other systemic diseases.

6. cost savings

In the long run, prevention is always more cost-effective than treatment. Regular dental cleaning can avoid expensive treatments that can result from neglect.

How natural teeth cleaning differs from conventional methods

In the world of oral care, there are constant ups and downs of trends and technologies. But one thing remains constant: the need to keep our teeth and gums healthy. But how do we achieve that? Traditional and natural approaches offer different methods and philosophies. Let's shed some light on the differences between these two paradigms.

1. ingredients and ingredients

- Traditional dental care: It often relies on a number of chemicals, including fluorides, artificial sweeteners and foaming agents such as sodium lauryl sulfate. These ingredients have specific functions, such as preventing tooth decay or providing a refreshing taste.
- Natural dental care: Here, everything revolves around the use of natural ingredients such as baking soda, coconut oil or essential oils. The idea is that nature itself often

provides solutions for our health needs without the need to resort to synthetic ingredients.

2. philosophy and approach

- Traditional dental care: It focuses mainly on combating problems after they have occurred, e.g. by removing plaque or fighting bacteria.
- Natural dental care: It takes a proactive approach that aims to strengthen oral health through preventive measures by keeping the oral microbiome in balance and providing the body with the necessary nutrients.

3. side effects and environmental impact

- Traditional dental care: Some of the chemicals used in traditional dental care products can cause irritation or allergies for some people. In addition, disposable toothbrushes and plastic packaging contribute to environmental problems.
- Natural dental care: It often uses environmentally friendly packaging and promotes sustainable practices. Since the ingredients are natural, allergic reactions or side effects are usually less common.

Example of a fictitious user: Lena

Lena has always had sensitive gums and was constantly on the lookout for a toothpaste that didn't burn or irritate. After switching to a natural toothpaste containing aloe vera and chamomile, she experienced significant relief and felt more comfortable brushing her teeth.

4. costs and availability

- Traditional dental care: These products are widely available in most drugstores and supermarkets. They are often cheaper because they are produced in large quantities.
- Natural dental care: It can be more expensive because the ingredients are often organic or of higher quality. But many argue that the extra cost is justified by the health benefits and lack of side effects.

Different techniques of natural teeth cleaning

1. oil pulling

Oil pulling is an ancient Ayurvedic technique that has been practiced for centuries. It involves rinsing the mouth with a tablespoon of oil, usually coconut or sesame oil, for about 15-20 minutes and then spitting the oil out. This method is said to draw toxins from the mouth and provide deep cleansing.

Advantages:

- Removal of harmful bacteria and plaque.
- Reduced gum inflammation.
- Natural whitening of the teeth.

Application:

Choose a cold-pressed, organic oil. Put a tablespoon in your mouth and rinse without swallowing. After 15-20 minutes, spit out and rinse with warm water.

2. use of baking soda (baking powder)

Baking soda, commonly known as baking powder, is often used as a natural tooth cleaning and whitening agent. It can serve as a gentle abrasive that removes stains from the tooth surface.

Advantages:

- Removal of surface stains.
- Neutralizes bad breath.

- Helps restore oral pH balance.

Application:

Moisten your toothbrush and dip it lightly in baking soda. Brush your teeth as usual, but be careful not to irritate the gums. Do not use daily so as not to damage tooth enamel.

3. herbal tinctures and rinses

Many herbs have antimicrobial and anti-inflammatory properties that make them ideal ingredients for natural mouthwashes. Some common herbs are sage, myrrh and echinacea.

Advantages:

- Fights bacteria and germs.
- Provides a soothing effect on inflamed or irritated gums.
- Freshens the breath.

Application:

Prepare a herbal tea with the selected herbs. Let it cool and use it as a mouthwash. Alternatively, you can buy ready-made herbal tinctures in pharmacies or health food stores.

Practical example: Emma

Emma, an avid hiker, always had problems with inflamed gums after long camping trips. After hearing about the benefits of herbal rinses, she began rinsing with an Echinacea decoction after every outdoor meal. Within a couple of weeks, she noticed a marked improvement in the health of her gums and vowed never to go back to traditional mouthwashes.

These are just three of the many natural techniques for cleaning teeth. In the following sections, we will delve further into the variety of these methods. It is important to note that everyone is different. What works for one person may not be ideal for another. Therefore, it is advisable to try different techniques and see which one suits you best.

4. activated carbon

Activated charcoal has gained popularity in recent years, especially for its ability to reduce discoloration on teeth. The porous structure of activated carbon attracts and removes impurities and stains from the teeth.

Advantages:

- Helps to whiten teeth.
- Eliminates bad breath.
- Binds toxins and bacteria.

Application:

Use a special toothpaste with activated charcoal or sprinkle a pinch of activated charcoal powder on your toothbrush. Brush gently and rinse thoroughly. This method should not be used daily.

5. miswak branches

Miswak, also known as "toothbrush tree", is a traditional cleaning instrument from the Middle East and Asia. It is a branch whose end is fanned out into bristles. It contains natural sources of fluoride and other minerals that contribute to the health of the teeth.

Advantages:

- Environmentally friendly and biodegradable.
- Can be used anywhere and without toothpaste.
- Strengthens the gums and prevents tooth decay.

Application:

Chew the end of the miswak branch until it splits into bristles. Brush your teeth with gentle movements. Rinse the miswak after use and store it in a dry place.

6. sea salt rinses

Salt has natural antiseptic properties, and sea salt contains an abundance of minerals that can benefit oral health.

Advantages:

- Prevents the growth of harmful bacteria.
- May reduce gingivitis.
- Neutralizes bad breath.

Application:

Dissolve one teaspoon of sea salt in a glass of warm water. Rinse the mouth with the solution for 30 seconds to one minute and then spit out.

Field report: Leo

Leo, a teacher from Munich, has always had sensitive gums. When he learned about the benefits of sea salt rinsing, he decided to give it a try. To his surprise, within a few weeks he noticed that his gums became less sensitive and more robust. He incorporated the sea salt rinse into his daily routine and was pleased with the visible results.

The beauty of natural teeth cleaning techniques is the variety of methods available. Depending on individual needs and preferences, one can choose the method that suits best. The range of techniques shows that nature has provided us with effective means of oral care without relying on chemical products.

7. green tea

Green tea contains polyphenols that can reduce harmful oral bacteria.

Advantages:

- Protects against caries.
- Fights bad breath.
- Reduces gingivitis.

Application:

Drink green tea regularly or rinse your mouth with green tea after drinking.

8. medicinal herbs and plants

Some medicinal herbs, such as sage and thyme, have antibacterial properties that can be useful in natural teeth cleaning.

Advantages:

- Prevents gingivitis.
- Reduces plaque formation.
- Fights harmful bacteria.

Application:

Crush the herbs into a paste and apply it with a toothbrush. Alternatively, you can make a tea from the herbs and rinse with it.

Field report: Mira

Mira, a dancer from Berlin, suffered from frequent mouth ulcers and gum problems. After incorporating sage into her daily tooth-cleaning routine, she noticed a significant improvement. The ulcers occurred less frequently, and her gums were healthier and less irritated.

The final part of this segment on natural tooth cleaning highlights the range of techniques available. Whether you choose a single method or combine several, these natural approaches can provide effective alternatives to commercial products while reducing environmental impact.

Instructions for making natural toothpastes and mouthwashes yourself

Natural toothpaste from coconut oil and turmeric

Ingredients:

- 2 tablespoons coconut oil
- 1 teaspoon turmeric powder
- A few drops of peppermint oil for the freshness kick

Preparation:

- Warm the coconut oil slightly in a water bath until it becomes liquid.
- Add the turmeric powder and stir well.
- Add a few drops of peppermint oil and stir again.
- Pour the mixture into a clean jar and leave to cool.

Usage: Use like a normal toothpaste. Turmeric is known for its anti-inflammatory properties, while coconut oil is antibacterial.

Natural mouthwash with sage and tea tree oil

Ingredients:

- 1 cup water
- 1 teaspoon sage leaves (fresh or dried)
- 2-3 drops tea tree oil

Preparation:

Bring water to a boil.

Add sage leaves and simmer for 5-10 minutes.

Remove the pot from the heat and let the liquid cool.

Pour the liquid through a sieve to remove the sage leaves.

Add a few drops of tea tree oil and stir well.

Usage: Use as a mouth rinse after brushing teeth. Do not swallow. Sage has antibacterial properties and can help keep gums healthy, while tea tree oil is a natural antiseptic.

Experience report: Tim

Tim, an avid backpacker, always had trouble finding eco-friendly dental care products while on the road. During a stay in a remote village in Asia, he learned about natural toothpaste made from coconut oil and turmeric and was thrilled with its effectiveness. When he returned, he experimented further and made his own natural dental care products. His teeth felt cleaner, and he appreciated the idea of not harming the environment.

Natural activated charcoal toothpaste

Ingredients:

- 1 teaspoon of activated charcoal powder (from the pharmacy or drugstore)
- 2 tablespoons coconut oil
- A few drops of lemon essential oil

Preparation:

- Melt the coconut oil slightly until it has a creamy consistency.
- Add activated carbon powder and mix well.
- Add a few drops of lemon essential oil for freshness and mix well again.
- Store in a clean jar or container.

Usage: Use like regular toothpaste. The activated charcoal can help remove stains and whiten teeth, while the lemon oil provides a fresh taste.

Natural mouthwash with green tea and cloves

Ingredients:

- 1 cup water
- 1 bag green tea
- 3-4 cloves

Preparation:

Bring water to a boil.

Add green tea bags and cloves.

Allow to infuse for 5 minutes.

Remove the tea bag and pour the liquid through a sieve to remove the cloves.

Allow to cool.

Usage: Use as a mouth rinse. The green tea contains antioxidants that can support oral health, and the cloves have analgesic and antibacterial effects.

Field report: Marlene

Marlene, a yoga teacher with a penchant for sustainability, was looking for ways to make her everyday life plastic-free. At a workshop, she learned about the benefits of activated charcoal and decided to create her own toothpaste. Not only did she appreciate the efficiency of homemade toothpaste, but she was impressed by the simplicity of the process and the ability to add her own touch. The green tea mouthwash became her daily ritual, and she noticed an improvement in the health of her gums in just a few weeks.

Natural alternatives to dental floss and interdental brushes

Miswak branches

Origin and history:

Miswak twigs, also known as Siwak or Sewak, come from the root wood of the Salvadora persica tree. For over 7000 years, people in Asia, the Middle East and Africa have used miswak as a natural toothbrush.

Advantages:

Contains natural fluorides, silicates and selenium compounds that strengthen teeth.

The fibers of the twig can be used to gently clean the interdental spaces.

Has antibacterial properties and fights tooth decay.

Usage:

- Cut off one end of the miswak twig about 1 cm and peel off the bark.
- Soak the exposed end for a few minutes until soft.
- Fluff the fibers by chewing.
- Rub against the teeth in a brushing motion and also gently clean the interdental spaces.

Neem branches

Origin and history:

Neem twigs come from the neem tree (Azadirachta indica). In India and other parts of Asia, it has been a tradition for centuries to use neem branches for oral care.

Advantages:

Has antibacterial and anti-inflammatory properties.

Helps prevent bleeding and inflammation of the gums.

Can reduce plaque and prevent tooth decay.

Usage:

Break off a small piece of neem branch.

Chew the end until it separates into fibers.

Use like a toothbrush and make sure that the interdental spaces are also reached.

Bamboo toothpick

Origin and history:

Bamboo toothpicks have been used for centuries in many Asian countries such as Japan and China. Bamboo has a natural strength and flexibility that makes it an ideal choice for oral care.

Advantages:

Bamboo is biodegradable and environmentally friendly.

It is naturally antimicrobial, which means that it does not easily accumulate bacteria.

Smooth, rounded edges that do not injure the gums.

Usage:

Simply use like a traditional toothpick, taking care to be gentle and not injure the gums.

Coconut oil pulling

Origin and history:

Oil pulling is an ancient Ayurvedic technique of rinsing oil in the mouth to remove toxins and promote oral health. Coconut oil has gained popularity in recent years because it is rich in lauric acid, which has antibacterial properties.

Advantages:

Can help reduce harmful bacteria in the mouth.

Promotes whiter teeth and fresher breath.

May reduce gingivitis and bleeding gums.

Usage:

Put a tablespoon of coconut oil in your mouth.

Swish the oil back and forth in your mouth for 15-20 minutes without swallowing.

Then spit out and rinse the mouth with warm water.

The journey of Lena

At a yoga retreat in Sri Lanka, Lena was introduced to coconut oil pulling. At first, she couldn't imagine that a simple oil could have so many benefits. But after trying it for a few days, she noticed how much cleaner and fresher her mouth felt. Her teeth appeared brighter, and the bleeding gums that had plagued her every morning for years were gone. Inspired by the experience, she made it a habit to incorporate oil pulling into her morning routine, and she has never regretted it. It was a powerful example to her of how powerful and effective natural methods can be.

How to build a natural teeth cleaning routine

1. develop the right attitude:

A natural teeth cleaning routine doesn't start with the products you use, but with your mindset. Recognize the value of natural ingredients and their benefits to your overall health and well-being.

2. create a daily ritual:

Consciously set aside time each morning and evening for your dental cleaning routine. A ritual rather than a chore can make all the difference in your motivation and consistency.

3. choose natural toothpaste:

Either buy one that doesn't contain artificial additives, or make your own. A simple recipe includes coconut oil, baking soda and a few drops of peppermint oil.

4. consider oil pulling:

As mentioned earlier, coconut oil pulling has many oral health benefits. Incorporate this ritual into your routine a few times a week.

5. do not use traditional dental floss:

Look for alternatives like silk or bamboo toothpicks that are bio-degradable and gentler on gums.

6. use a natural mouthwash:

Forget mouthwashes that contain alcohol. A mix of warm water, sea salt and a few drops of tea tree oil can be just as effective.

7. keep an eye on nutrition:

A healthy diet plays a crucial role in the health of teeth and gums. Avoid too much sugar and go for foods rich in calcium and vitamin D.

8. regular checks:

Even if you use natural methods, you should have your teeth checked regularly by a dentist. He can give you feedback on your routine and make sure everything is in the best order.

9. continuing education:

The world of natural health and care is constantly changing. Stay up to date by reading books, taking online courses or attending workshops.

Laura's story

Laura has always been a fan of natural remedies. When she noticed how aggressive some commercial dental care products can be, she decided to create her own natural teeth cleaning routine. After a few months of experimenting and learning, she had found a system that worked for her. Her teeth felt cleaner, her breath was fresher, and she felt like she was doing something good for herself and the planet. She never looked back.

4. Natural teeth whitening

For many, seeing a brilliant white in the mirror when we smile is a sign of health and beauty. But it is not uncommon for our teeth to take on a different color over time. Here we explore the reasons behind this discoloration.

1. succumb to the passage of time:

Just as our skin changes over the years, so do our teeth. The dentin, the inner, naturally yellowish material of the tooth, becomes denser over time, while the outer enamel becomes thinner. This combination results in a less radiant white.

2. love goes through the stomach, but what sticks to the teeth?

Whether it's the morning coffee or the glass of red wine in the evening - many of our favorite drinks contain color pigments that can stick to the teeth and discolor them.

3. smoke signals:

Cigarette smoke contains chemicals that are not only harmful to our health, but also to our teeth. Nicotine and tar can cause yellow or even brown stains that are difficult to remove.

4. the attack of the acid monsters:

Acidic foods and beverages attack tooth enamel. This erosion process makes the teeth more susceptible to discoloration, as they become more porous and absorb stains more easily.

5. genes also play a role:

Just like our eye color or hair color, the natural color and texture of our teeth is also partly genetically determined.

6. medical side effects:

Some medications and medical treatments, such as chemotherapy, can cause discoloration of the teeth. These drugs either directly affect the enamel or change the flow of saliva, which in turn affects the teeth.

Difference between natural and artificial teeth whitening

Everyone wants a bright smile, but the way to achieve this goal can vary. On the cosmetics shelf, you'll find a variety of products for whitening teeth, and there are just as many home remedies circulating that are supposed to help you achieve a brighter smile. But what actually distinguishes these methods?

1. natural teeth whitening: back to nature

Active principles: Natural teeth whitening mainly uses natural ingredients such as baking soda, coconut oil or strawberry pulp. These ingredients often contain slightly abrasive or enzymatic components that can remove surface discolorations.

Gentleness: Since natural remedies often contain less aggressive ingredients, they are usually gentler on teeth and gums. However, this does not mean that they are always harmless. Excessive abrasiveness can damage tooth enamel.

Time span: Natural whitening methods often require patience and regular use over a long period of time.

2. artificial teeth whitening: the power of science

Active principles: These often involve chemical processes. Bleaching products containing hydrogen peroxide or carbamide peroxide penetrate the tooth and decompose the discolorations from the inside.

Efficiency: Artificial methods usually show faster results than natural ones. With professional treatments at the dentist, significant changes can be noticed after just one session.

Safety: While products used by professionals are safe when used properly, over-the-counter products or misapplied remedies can cause tooth sensitivity or gum irritation.

3. cost and availability

Natural teeth whitening: One of the great advantages of natural methods is their cost-effectiveness. Many of the ingredients needed can already be found in the kitchen or can be purchased at a fraction of the price of professional whitening. There is also a certain satisfaction in preparing your own mixture of natural ingredients.

Artificial tooth whitening: Professional whitening methods or specialized kits can be expensive. Their prices vary depending on the brand, quality and concentration of active ingredients. But they also usually promise more visible and often longer-lasting results.

4. durability and maintenance

Natural methods: Although often described as gentler, some natural whiteners can wear away tooth enamel over time, especially if used too frequently. This can lead to permanent sensitivity. Results are often subtle and can last longer with proper aftercare.

Artificial methods: Despite their efficiency, chemical whiteners can also damage tooth enamel if used incorrectly or too frequently. However, their results are usually longer lasting, and regular refreshing is recommended.

5. side effects and risks

Natural methods: The most common side effects include temporary tooth sensitivity and possible erosion of tooth enamel with excessive use.

Artificial methods: Here, side effects such as tooth sensitivity, gum irritation and, in rare cases, chemical burns may occur.

Tom's experience:

Tom, an avid coffee drinker, was concerned about the discoloration of his teeth. He started using a natural method that included coconut oil. While he noticed minimal whitening, he looked for something more potent. A drugstore whitening kit provided more impressive results, but Tom also experienced tooth sensitivity. The experience taught him that both natural and artificial methods have their own pros and cons, and that it's important to be well-informed before making a decision.

Foods and habits that help whiten teeth naturally

1. the crunchy duo: apples and carrots

Crunchy foods like apples and carrots act like a natural brush when chewed. Due to their firm structure, they help clean the surface of the teeth and remove plaque, which is often responsible for discoloration. At the same time, they stimulate the gums through chewing, which promotes oral health.

Tip: A crisp apple after a meal can work wonders, especially if you don't have the opportunity to brush your teeth right away.

2. strawberries - sweet and useful

Strawberries contain malic acid, a natural fruit acid that can help remove surface stains. But be careful: too much acid can damage tooth enamel. Therefore, this method should be used in moderation.

A simple recipe: Crush a strawberry and mix it with a pinch of baking soda. Apply the paste to your teeth and leave it on for a few minutes. Then rinse and brush thoroughly to remove any residue.

3. the straw trick

Dark beverages such as coffee, tea or red wine are often the culprits for tooth discoloration. A simple trick to reduce direct contact with teeth is to use a straw. This allows the drinks to go directly into the throat and bypass the teeth for the most part.

4. the milk does it

Dairy products such as yogurt, cheese and milk are rich in calcium, which strengthens and protects tooth enamel. Strong enamel is less susceptible to discoloration. In addition, some proteins in milk, called caseins, bind colorants from food, preventing them from being deposited on teeth.

5. xylitol chewing gum: The sweet cleanser

Xylitol is a natural sweetener found in some chewing gums. It has the advantage of fighting bacteria that cause tooth decay. Chewing xylitol gum also promotes saliva production, which helps neutralize and rinse acids and food debris from the teeth.

6. green, green, green tea

Although teas are generally considered to cause tooth discoloration, green tea has the advantage of containing fluoride. Fluoride can help strengthen and protect tooth enamel. However, it is important to enjoy green tea in moderation and rinse the mouth with water after consumption.

7. crunchy celery

Similar to apples and carrots, celery has a textured texture that "scrubs" the teeth when chewed. Its fibers act like a natural toothbrush that can remove plaque and stains.

8. broccoli: the green shield

Broccoli eaten raw forms a kind of protective film on the teeth when chewed. This film can help prevent discoloration caused by other foods. In addition, broccoli is rich in iron, which protects tooth enamel and reduces the adhesion of harmful bacteria and acids.

9. nuts and seeds for exfoliation

Nuts and seeds have abrasive properties that can help remove plaque and stains on the teeth. Almonds, walnuts and sunflower seeds are particularly recommended here. When chewed, they break into small particles that provide a kind of micro-peeling for the teeth.

10. drinking water: the universal cleaner

Drinking water regularly, especially after consuming staining foods or beverages, helps rinse the mouth and prevent discoloration. Water also neutralizes the acids that can attack tooth enamel.

11. juicy strawberries

While many fruits can contribute to tooth discoloration, strawberries are a natural whitener thanks to their high vitamin C content. They help remove plaque, which can lead to tooth discoloration. A bonus? The malicide in strawberries also contributes to whitening. However, it is recommended that you rinse your mouth thoroughly after eating them.

12. vitamin rich vegetables

Vegetables like peppers and tomatoes, which are rich in vitamin C, can keep gums healthy and prevent the development of periodontal disease. Healthy gums contribute to an overall brighter smile.

13. dairy products - bright smile thanks to calcium

Milk, cheese and yogurt not only contain calcium and phosphate, which strengthen tooth enamel, but also help neutralize the pH in the mouth, protecting teeth from acid attacks.

14. oil pulling with coconut oil

An ancient Ayurvedic method for improving oral health is oil pulling. This involves swishing a tablespoon of oil, preferably coconut oil, back and forth in the mouth for 10-15 minutes. Many people report that this method leads to whiter teeth and reduces bacteria in the mouth.

15. avoid coloring foods and beverages

Last but not least, prevention is one of the best ways to maintain a bright smile. This means limiting the consumption of coffee, tea, red wine and other highly staining foods and beverages, or at least rinsing the mouth with water after consuming them.

Elena's Insider Tip:

Elena, an avid dancer and fitness enthusiast, always paid close attention to her diet. However, when she learned about the brightening properties of some foods, she consciously integrated them into her diet. Soon, she noticed not only a stronger body image, but also a brighter smile that she proudly displayed on the dance floor.

Instructions for various natural teeth whitening techniques

1. baking powder and water:

A classic home remedy that can be found in many kitchens.

Ingredients:

- 1 teaspoon baking powder
- A few drops of water

Instruction:

Mix the baking soda with the water drops to form a paste.

Use the mixture like a normal toothpaste.

Brush teeth for a maximum of 2 minutes and then rinse thoroughly.

Do not use this method more than once a week to avoid damaging the enamel.

2. activated carbon for a sparkling smile:

Activated charcoal can effectively pull stains from teeth and make them look brighter.

Ingredients:

1 capsule of activated charcoal (available in any drugstore)

Instruction:

- Open the activated charcoal capsule and put the contents on your toothbrush.
- Brush your teeth gently, making sure to reach all areas.
- After 2 minutes, rinse thoroughly.
- This procedure should be used no more than once a week.

3. coconut oil pulling - tradition meets modern oral care:

Coconut oil is not only known for its moisturizing properties, but it can also help whiten teeth.

Ingredients:

1-2 tablespoons virgin coconut oil

Instruction:

Put the coconut oil in your mouth.

Pull and push the oil through your teeth for 10-20 minutes.

Spit the oil out afterwards (not down the drain as it can clog).

Rinse with warm water and then brush teeth as usual.

The trick with the sage:

Sophie, a garden lover, discovered the benefit of sage leaves for a whiter smile. Every time she harvested fresh sage from her garden, she gently rubbed a leaf over her teeth. The results were amazing, and soon she swapped her regular toothpaste for her new natural method.

4. strawberry salt paste - A sweet secret:

The fruit acid in strawberries can help remove tooth discoloration, while salt acts as a natural abrasive.

Ingredients:

2-3 ripe strawberries

A pinch of sea salt

Instruction:

- Mash the strawberries in a bowl.
- Add the sea salt and mix to form a paste.
- Apply to teeth and leave for 3-5 minutes.
- Rinse thoroughly and brush teeth as usual.

This method should be used only once a week, so as not to damage the enamel.

5. apple cider vinegar rinse:

Apple cider vinegar contains acids that can dissolve stains. However, you should be careful with it so as not to damage the enamel.

Ingredients:

1 part apple cider vinegar

2 parts water

Instruction:

Mix the apple cider vinegar with water.

Use the solution as a mouthwash, rinse with it for about one minute.

Then rinse thoroughly with water and brush your teeth.

Application maximum once a week.

6. banana peel - use the inside:

The inside of a banana peel contains substances that can be helpful in whitening teeth.

Instruction:

- After eating a banana, take the inside of the peel.
- Gently rub the inside of the bowl over your teeth.
- Leave on for about 10 minutes and then brush teeth thoroughly.

Use daily for best results.

The secret of turmeric:

In a small kitchen in a village nestled at the foot of the mountains, Clara set out to create a special toothpaste made from turmeric, a well-known spice with anti-inflammatory properties. Some of her friends were skeptical, but after a few weeks they were surprised when Clara's teeth became visibly brighter. It became a beloved beauty secret in her village.

7. lemon and baking soda mask:

The combination of lemon juice and baking soda can act as a natural bleaching agent.

Ingredients:

Juice from half a lemon

One teaspoon baking powder

Instruction:

Mix the lemon juice with the baking soda to make a thick paste.

Apply the mixture to your teeth and leave it on for no longer than a minute.

Then rinse thoroughly and brush teeth.

Use no more than once a month, as the acid can damage tooth enamel.

8. activated carbon - A dark secret for brighter teeth:

Activated charcoal can bind toxins and stains for brighter teeth.

Ingredients:

Activated charcoal capsule or powder

Instruction:

- Put a small amount of activated charcoal powder on your toothbrush.
- Gently brush your teeth with it for 2 minutes.
- Then rinse thoroughly and brush teeth with normal tooth-paste.

Apply once or twice a week.

9. coconut oil pulling:

Coconut oil contains lauric acid, which has antibacterial effects and can reduce plaque.

Ingredients:

1-2 tablespoons pure coconut oil

Instruction:

- Put the coconut oil in your mouth and "pull" it between your teeth.
- Continue for 15-20 minutes and then spit it out (not down the drain!).
- Rinse with warm water and brush teeth as usual.

Use daily for optimal results.

The saga of Rosalind and the olive oil:

Rosalind, an avid herbalist from a dreamy seaside village, discovered the tooth whitening properties of olive oil during her experiments with natural beauty products. She mixed the oil with a little salt and used the mixture as a toothpaste. The villagers were impressed with her radiant smile and soon many followed her example. The village became known for the healthy looking teeth of its inhabitants.

How to prevent discoloration through diet and lifestyle

A radiant smile is not only an expression of health and self-confidence, but it also reflects the care you give your body and especially your teeth. However, over time, discoloration can form on the teeth. Here are some useful tips to minimize such discoloration through a conscious diet and adapted lifestyle:

1. balanced diet:

Eating fresh fruits and vegetables not only promotes overall health, but also stimulates the production of saliva, which naturally helps keep the mouth clean.

2. drink wisely:

Tea, coffee, red wine and dark juices can cause discoloration. Consider rinsing your mouth with water or drinking through a straw after consuming such beverages to reduce direct contact with teeth.

3. beware of acidic foods and drinks:

Citrus fruits, vinegar or carbonated drinks can soften tooth enamel. After eating acidic foods, wait about 30 minutes before brushing your teeth to avoid additional enamel erosion.

4. reduction of sugar and sweets:

Bacteria in the mouth turn sugar into acid, which can attack tooth enamel. If you have eaten something sweet, you should rinse your mouth or brush your teeth afterwards.

5. refrain from smoking:

Nicotine is not only harmful to the lungs, but also a major cause of tooth discoloration. Therefore, giving up smoking can lead to a visible improvement in the appearance of the teeth.

6. regular oral hygiene:

Brushing twice a day, flossing and regular dental check-ups are essential to prevent tooth discoloration and disease.

The findings of Ferdinand the Fisherman:

Ferdinand, a prudent fisherman from a remote coastal village, noticed that despite his regular tea consumption, some of his friends had noticeably whiter teeth. When he inquired, one of the village elders told him the secret: they rinsed their mouths with fresh spring water after every cup of tea. Ferdinand took this ritual to heart and soon noticed an improvement. This simple remedy showed that often small changes in routine can have a big impact on the health and aesthetics of our teeth.

Testimonials from people who have used natural teeth whitening methods

Sophie's experience with baking powder:

Sophie, a young woman in her thirties, had always struggled with slightly yellowish discolored teeth. She stumbled across an article online describing the effects of baking soda as a natural teeth whitener and decided to try it out for herself. Once a week, she dipped her toothbrush in a small amount of baking soda and brushed her teeth with it. The change was remarkable after a few weeks. However, Sophie stressed that she did not use it daily so as not to damage the enamel. For her, it was a cost-effective method that she was happy to recommend, while advising everyone to do it wisely and keep an eye on their enamel.

Marco's adventure with coconut oil:

Marco, a fun-loving dancer, had heard about the "oil pulling" method with coconut oil. At first he was skeptical - how could oil whiten teeth? But his curiosity drove him to try it. Every morning, he put a tablespoon of coconut oil in his mouth and "pulled" it through his teeth for about 20 minutes before spitting it out and rinsing his mouth thoroughly with water. Not only did he notice a gradual whitening of his teeth, but also an overall fresher mouth-feel. For Marco, it was more than just a whitening method; it became a morning ritual that also helped him prepare for the day.

Lena's experience with strawberry paste:

Lena, a young mother and amateur gardener, read in an old gardening book about the natural whitening effect of strawberries. She mashed ripe strawberries into a paste, mixed it with half a teaspoon of baking soda and applied the mixture to her teeth. After five minutes, she rinsed her mouth. She used the strawberry paste twice a week and noticed a gentle whitening of her teeth after a month. Additionally, she loved the fresh strawberry flavor, which was an added bonus. However, Lena warned against using this method too often, as the acid in the strawberries could attack tooth enamel.

These stories show that natural methods of teeth whitening can certainly work. However, as with all things in life, it is important to be moderate and not lose sight of your own health.

Tom's experiment with activated carbon:

Tom's story began in a health store when he stumbled across activated charcoal capsules. He had read that activated charcoal can bind toxins and also help whiten teeth. After opening a capsule and putting the contents on his toothbrush, he carefully brushed his teeth with it. The results after a few weeks were amazing: his teeth became noticeably whiter. However, Tom stressed that it was important to rinse thoroughly afterwards to remove any charcoal residue and that application should be limited to once a week.

Isabella's discovery of apple cider vinegar:

Isabella, an avid cook, often used apple cider vinegar in her salad dressings. When she learned that it could also be used to whiten teeth, she was curious. She mixed water and apple cider vinegar in equal parts and used the solution as a mouth rinse. After a few weeks, she noticed that her teeth became brighter. However, she cautioned against keeping the vinegar in her mouth for too long, as the acid can damage tooth enamel. A quick rinse and then rinsing the mouth with clean water was the key to success for her.

Olivia's encounter with turmeric:

Olivia, a globetrotter, discovered the many benefits of turmeric during a trip to India. One of the locals recommended that she try turmeric as a natural teeth whitener. She was hesitant at first because the spice can leave intense yellow stains, but she was brave enough to try it. She made a paste of turmeric powder and water and brushed her teeth with it. To her surprise, after several applications, the results were impressive without staining the teeth. She recommended this method to others, but advised caution when handling turmeric because of its staining power on clothing and skin.

Each of these reports not only highlights the effectiveness of natural teeth whitening methods, but also emphasizes the importance of caution and regularity in their use. It is impressive how nature offers us so many wonderful solutions, if we only know where to look.

Luke and the coconut oil pulling:

Luke came across the traditional method of oil pulling during a trip through Southeast Asia. Soon coconut oil pulling became a regular part of his morning routine. Every morning, he put a tablespoon of coconut oil in his mouth and "pulled" it through his teeth for about 20 minutes before spitting it out. The result? Fresher breath and noticeably whiter teeth after a few months.

Lukas is convinced that coconut oil pulling not only whitened his teeth, but also kept his gums healthy.

Melanie's experience with strawberry baking soda paste:

Melanie, a mother of three, was constantly looking for quick and natural home remedies. One recipe she tried was a paste made from crushed strawberries and baking soda. She applied the mixture to her teeth a few times a week and left it on for five minutes. Melanie noticed that this mixture not only counteracted discoloration, but also freshened her breath. One tip she passed along was to rinse thoroughly after application and brush her teeth with plain water to remove any residue.

Jasmin's discovery of the banana peel method:

During a conversation in an environmental group, Jasmin learned about the amazing use of banana peels for dental care. Curious, she gently rubbed the inside of the peel over her teeth after eating a banana. After several weeks of use, she noticed a subtle but noticeable whitening of her teeth. Not only was this an environmentally friendly method because it reduced waste, but she found it reassuring that she had used a completely chemical-free method.

These experiences show that there is an abundance of natural remedies that are not only effective, but also environmentally friendly and inexpensive. While results may vary, the common denominator is that patience and regularity are essential to achieve visible results.

5. Healthy gums and oral flora

One thing is clear: when we think about oral health, we often tend to focus exclusively on our teeth. The bright smile, the flawless row of teeth - all of this is the focus of our attention. But far from this spotlight, the gums play an inconspicuous but absolutely central role.

A natural protective wall:

The gums act as a barrier, protecting the roots of our teeth from harmful bacteria. Without this covering, microorganisms could easily invade the dental area and cause infections or damage that can lead to tooth loss.

An early warning system:

Bleeding gums are not only an indication of possible gingivitis, but can also be a warning sign of other health problems, such as diabetes or heart disease. Healthy gums are pink and do not bleed during normal brushing or eating.

The connection with the bone:

The gums and the underlying jawbone are inextricably linked. Weakened or diseased gums can cause the jawbone to recede. This in turn can affect the stability of the teeth and lead to their loosening or loss.

A mirror of general well-being:

Stress, poor diet or lack of oral care can affect the gums. Conversely, unhealthy gums can lead to bad breath and affect self-esteem. Care of the gums thus contributes significantly to our general well-being.

An influencing factor for the aesthetic aspect:

In addition to its purely functional role, the gums also influence how our smile is perceived. Healthy, even gums give the smile an aesthetic balance and complete the overall appearance.

In summary, the health of our gums has a profound effect on overall oral health. It is the invisible foundation that supports the beauty and function of our smile. Therefore, it should receive as much attention in our daily oral care as our teeth themselves. It is a delicate part of our body that deserves care and respect.

How to recognize and prevent gum disease

Recognizing warning signs: The key to prevention

One of the main problems with gum disease is that it is often painless at first and therefore easy to overlook. Nevertheless, there are signs that can signal to us that something is wrong.

The sooner you recognize these signs, the better you can treat them and prevent worse problems.

1. bleeding gums:

It is a common myth that occasional bleeding gums while brushing or flossing is normal. It isn't. Even mild bleeding can indicate the onset of gingivitis.

2. changes in the color of the gums:

Healthy gums have a pale pink color. If your gums appear red or even purple, this could be a sign of inflammation.

3. swollen gums:

Swelling is often a sign of inflammation. If you notice that areas of your gums are swollen or tender, this is a clear warning signal.

4. recession of the gums:

Do you feel that your teeth look "longer" than before? This could indicate that your gums are receding, which in turn may be a symptom of advanced gum disease.

5. bad breath:

Constant bad breath or a foul taste in the mouth can be signs of the presence of harmful bacteria that cause gum disease.

First steps for prevention

1. optimal oral hygiene:

Eliminating plaque by brushing and flossing regularly is the first step to preventing gum disease. Invest in a good toothbrush and change it every 3-4 months.

2. regular visits to the dentist:

Only a dentist can really detect the first signs of gum disease, especially in areas that are difficult to see or clean. A regular check-up, ideally every six months, is essential.

3. healthy diet:

A diet rich in vitamins C and E can help keep gums healthy. Both vitamins have anti-inflammatory properties and play a role in tissue repair.

At its core, it's about being vigilant and proactive. Recognizing the first warning signs and taking preventive measures can be key to keeping your smile bright and your gums healthy.

Other signs of gum disease

1. loosening of the teeth:

A firm bite is a sign of healthy teeth and gums. If you notice that your teeth are loosening or shifting, this can be an alarm signal.

2. sensitivity to heat and cold:

If your gums are inflamed, this can lead to greater sensitivity to temperature differences, especially with hot or cold drinks and foods.

3. painful chewing:

When chewing becomes a painful affair, it is often a warning sign of gingivitis or a deeper infection.

Understanding the root causes

In most cases, gum disease begins with the accumulation of plaque, a sticky film of bacteria. If plaque is not removed regularly, it can become tartar, which further damages the gums.

Smoking is a major cause of gum disease and can slow down the healing process after treatment. Similarly, diseases that affect the immune system, such as diabetes, can increase the risk of infections in the mouth.

Hormonal changes in women can make the gums more sensitive and more easily inflamed. These include puberty, menstruation, pregnancy and menopause.

Prevention strategies for healthy gums

1. the correct technique for brushing teeth:

It is not only important how often, but also how you brush your teeth. Gentle, circular movements are effective and prevent the gums from receding or being injured.

2. mouthwash:

Antiseptic mouthwash can help reduce bacteria and thus minimize plaque formation. However, it is important to note that not all mouthwash products are the same. Some may even contain alcohol, which can dry out gums. It's worth choosing a mouthwash specifically designed to strengthen gums and fight bacteria.

3. a healthy lifestyle:

A balanced diet, physical activity and avoiding tobacco products can contribute significantly to the prevention of gum disease. Reducing sugary drinks and snacks should also not be forgotten.

The progressive stages of gum disease

1. gingivitis (inflammation of the gums):

The earliest stage of gum disease, characterized by red, swollen gums that can bleed easily. Fortunately, gingivitis is reversible because the bone and surrounding tissues are not yet affected.

2. periodontitis:

If gingivitis is not treated, it can progress to periodontitis. Here, the gum pockets begin to deepen, giving bacteria access to the roots of the teeth and the jawbone. This can lead to tooth loss.

3. advanced periodontitis:

In this final stage of the disease, the fibers and bones that support the teeth are severely damaged. The teeth may shift or become loose and may need to be removed.

Specialized cleaning and treatment

For people who already show signs of gum disease, professional dental cleaning may be essential. This involves removing plaque and tartar above and below the gumline.

In more severe cases, scaling and root planing treatment may be required. This is a deep cleaning that removes bacteria and rough tartar from the roots of the teeth.

Natural home remedies for healthy gums

1. salt water rinses:

A warm salt water rinse can help reduce swelling and kill bacteria that can cause gum problems.

2. aloe vera:

The gel-like substance from the aloe vera plant has anti-inflammatory and healing properties that can help with gum inflammation.

3. green tea:

Green tea contains antioxidants that can fight inflammation and keep gums healthy.

Final thoughts

Detecting and preventing gum disease requires a certain level of awareness and commitment to daily oral care. Regular dental exams and professional cleanings can detect and treat deeper problems early. Combine this with some of the natural home remedies mentioned above, and you have a recipe for a lifetime of healthy smiles.

Natural remedies and practices for the care of the gums

Healthy gums are the foundation for strong teeth and a bright smile. Instead of relying solely on commercial products, you can harness the power of nature to strengthen and protect your gums. Discover these traditional and natural methods to care for and strengthen your gums.

1. oil pulling with coconut oil:

This time-honored Ayurvedic practice consists of swishing a tablespoon of coconut oil in the mouth for about 15-20 minutes. Oil pulling can help remove harmful bacteria from the mouth and prevent gingivitis. Coconut oil is also known for its antimicrobial properties.

2. neem:

Neem leaves and bark have been known for centuries in traditional medicine for their antiseptic and anti-inflammatory properties. A neem leaf tea can be used as a mouthwash to strengthen the gums and fight bad breath.

3. green tea:

A daily cup of green tea can work wonders. The antioxidants it contains, especially catechin, can reduce inflammation in the gums and support dental health.

4. chamomile tea rinse:

Chamomile is known for its soothing and anti-inflammatory properties. A rinse with cooled chamomile tea can help reduce gum swelling and irritation.

5. vitamin rich diet:

Vitamins, especially vitamin C and K, are essential for gum health. Citrus fruits, broccoli and peppers are rich in vitamin C, while dark green leafy vegetables are an excellent source of vitamin K.

6. myrrh tincture:

Used in traditional Chinese medicine, myrrh can serve as a natural mouthwash. It can help with gingivitis and has soothing properties.

7. xylitol gum:

Although not technically "natural," xylitol can help slow the growth of harmful bacteria in the mouth. It is derived from birch bark and can balance the pH level in the mouth.

8. regular brushing and flossing:

It may seem obvious, but using a soft toothbrush and flossing daily is one of the best ways to prevent gum disease. The

natural gum massaging experience of brushing promotes circu-
lation and health.

9. aloe vera gel:

Another soothing agent is the gel of the aloe vera plant. It can
be applied directly to the gums to soothe irritation and inflammation.

The role of oral flora in dental health

In the hidden corners of our mouths exists a vibrant, pulsating
city of microscopic inhabitants: the oral flora. It is a community of
billions of microorganisms that populate our oral cavity. But what
exactly do these tiny creatures do in our mouths, and what role
do they play in the health of our teeth and gums?

1. microscopic inhabitants with macroscopic influence:

Our oral flora consists of bacteria, viruses, fungi and protozoa.
Of the more than 700 identified species of bacteria in the mouth,
many are harmless or even beneficial, while others can be potentially harmful.

2. the protectors:

Good bacteria, often called probiotics, play an important role in
preventing disease. They do this by consuming nutrients that

would otherwise be available to harmful bacteria and by producing substances that inhibit the growth of harmful bacteria.

3. an imbalance leads to problems:

An imbalance or dysbiosis of the oral flora can lead to various oral health problems. Harmful bacteria can proliferate and lead to tooth decay, gingivitis and other oral infections.

4. pH value and bacteria:

The pH value in the mouth influences the growth of certain types of bacteria. An acidic pH favors cariogenic (caries-causing) bacteria, while a neutral pH promotes the growth of beneficial bacteria.

5. plaque and bacteria:

Plaque is a biofilm composed of bacteria, saliva proteins and food residues. The bacteria it contains produce acids that can attack tooth enamel. Regular removal of plaque is therefore essential to maintain dental health.

6. entry port for the body:

The oral cavity is not only important for our dental health. Harmful microorganisms from the mouth can enter the bloodstream and affect other parts of the body, increasing the risk of cardiovascular disease, diabetes and other conditions.

7. probiotics for the mouth:

There is growing evidence that probiotics taken orally can promote not only gut health but also oral health. These "good" bacteria compete with harmful bacteria for resources and can thus
restore the balance of the oral flora.

Graduation:

The oral flora is much more than just a bunch of bacteria in the
mouth; it is an essential part of our oral ecosystem. Understanding their function and influence allows us to make better deci-
sions regarding our oral care and overall health. So it is of ut-
most importance to give these tiny inhabitants the attention they
deserve.

Probiotics and prebiotics for healthy oral flora

When we think of probiotics and prebiotics, many of us think first
of the gut. But did you know that these two powerful partners
can also be crucial for a healthy oral flora? Let's dive into the
fascinating world of microorganisms and find out how these two
terms influence our oral microbiome.

1. probiotics - The good bacteria:

Probiotics are living microorganisms that, when taken in sufficient quantities, provide health benefits to the host. In the mouth, they act as natural defenders that help keep harmful bacteria at bay and restore the natural balance of oral flora.

Power of counterparts: Probiotic bacteria compete with harmful bacteria for the same food sources, reducing the growth of potentially harmful microbes.

Guardians of pH: Some probiotics produce substances that can neutralize the pH in the mouth, reducing the risk of tooth decay.

2. prebiotics - food for the good guys:

Prebiotics are non-digestible food components that promote the growth and activity of probiotic bacteria. They are, so to speak, the "food" for our good bacteria and help them to thrive and develop their protective properties.

Natural Boost: Eating prebiotic foods such as garlic, onions and asparagus can promote the growth of probiotic bacteria in the mouth.

Resist the bad guys: prebiotics ensure probiotic bacteria stay strong and healthy to effectively fight harmful bacteria.

3. the synergy of pro- and prebiotics:

Together, probiotics and prebiotics work hand in hand to maintain the microbial balance in the mouth. While probiotics form the front line in the defense, prebiotics provide them with the necessary energy to perform their task efficiently.

4. recommendations for everyday life:

To get the most out of probiotics and prebiotics, consider taking probiotic supplements or consuming foods rich in these valuable microorganisms, such as yogurt or sauerkraut. Likewise, you should incorporate prebiotic foods into your diet to support the growth and health of your probiotic bacteria.

Conclusion:

The healthy balance of oral flora is a crucial factor for overall oral health. Probiotics and prebiotics play an important role in maintaining and promoting this balance. By integrating these powerful microorganisms and their food sources into our daily lives, we can go one step further in keeping our teeth and gums healthy.

6. Prevention and natural treatment of oral diseases.

The mouth is much more than just the gateway to digestion; it is also a complex ecosystem in which both protective and harmful microorganisms coexist. However, mismanagement and neglect of oral care can lead to serious diseases. Below, we look at the three most common oral diseases and provide tips on how to avoid them.

1. caries - the secret destroyer:

Dental caries, also known as tooth decay, is one of the most common diseases worldwide. It occurs when acid-producing bacteria attack the tooth surface and weaken it.

Recognition: Early signs are white spots on the teeth, followed by small holes or discoloration.

Prevention: Regular and thorough dental care with fluoride toothpaste, limiting sugary snacks and drinks, and regular dental check-ups are essential.

2. gingivitis - the red alarm signal:

Gingivitis is an inflammation of the gums caused by plaque bacteria. Without treatment, it can lead to periodontitis.

Recognize: Symptoms include red, swollen gums and bleeding when brushing or flossing.

Prevention: Daily brushing and flossing, mouthwash, and regular dental cleanings can help prevent gingivitis.

3. periodontitis - the hidden enemy:

Periodontitis is an advanced form of gum inflammation that affects the jawbone and can eventually lead to tooth loss.

Recognize: Signs include deep gum pockets, receding gums, loose teeth and persistent bad breath.

Prevention: Early diagnosis and treatment of gingivitis, thorough cleaning routines and professional dental check-ups are essential.

Healthy habits for a healthy mouth:

Prevention is the key when it comes to oral diseases. Besides the above tips, you should also:

Use mouthwashes containing fluoride.

Clean the interdental spaces with interdental brushes or dental floss.

Prefer a low-sugar diet.

Visit the dentist regularly, not only in case of complaints.

Conclusion:

The health of your mouth often reflects the overall health of your body. A proactive approach to caring for your teeth and gums can not only keep your smile bright, but also prevent serious diseases. A healthy mouth is a happy mouth!

Natural remedies and practices for the prevention and treatment of oral diseases.

Long before the advent of modern medicine, our ancestors relied on the forces of nature to treat and prevent oral diseases. Many of these time-tested methods have withstood the test of time and continue to provide us with valuable solutions today. Let's dive into the world of natural remedies and practices:

1. oil pulling - Ancient Ayurvedic knowledge:

Oil pulling, especially with coconut oil, is an ancient method from Ayurveda. It is believed that swishing oil in the mouth removes harmful bacteria.

Application: Take one tablespoon of coconut oil and move it in the mouth for 15-20 minutes. Then spit out and rinse the mouth with warm water.

2. green tea - An antioxidant giant:

Green tea contains polyphenols that can inhibit the growth of bacteria that cause tooth decay.

Directions: Drink one to two cups of green tea daily, unsweetened, for maximum benefit.

3. aloe vera - the miracle gel:

Aloe vera has anti-inflammatory properties and can help with gingivitis.

Application: Apply Aloe Vera Gel directly to the affected area or use as a mouth rinse.

4. xylitol chewing gums - A natural enemy of bacteria:

Xylitol, a natural sugar alcohol, can reduce the growth of bacteria in the mouth.

Application: Chew xylitol gum after meals. It helps reduce acid production and remineralizes tooth enamel.

5. sage - A herb with history:

Sage has antibacterial properties that are useful in the treatment of gingivitis.

Application: Prepare a strong infusion of sage leaves and use as a mouthwash.

6. eat a diet rich in vitamins:

Vitamins, especially vitamin C and D, play a crucial role in the health of teeth and gums.

Directions: Supplement a balanced diet with fresh fruits, vegetables and fish oil. Deficiency can lead to bleeding gums and tooth loss.

7. proper brushing:

The most natural and effective remedy for oral diseases is brushing the teeth with a soft brush in circular movements.

Application: Brush thoroughly but gently at least twice a day, morning and evening.

Closing thought:

Although these natural remedies and practices provide valuable tools to prevent and treat oral diseases, they do not replace the need for regular dental checkups. It is important to take a balanced approach that integrates both modern and natural solutions to ensure the best oral health.

The role of nutrition in the prevention of oral diseases

It's often said, "You are what you eat." When it comes to the health of our mouths, this old saying couldn't be more apt. The way we eat has far-reaching effects on our oral health, from the strength of our tooth enamel to the health of our gums. Let's take a look at how our eating habits affect oral disease prevention.

1. foods rich in calcium:

Dairy products such as milk, yogurt and cheese are rich in calcium, which is essential for strong teeth and healthy gums.

2. foods with high water content:

Fruits and vegetables such as apples, cucumbers and celery not only help with hydration, but also clean the teeth and gums as you chew, reducing plaque buildup.

3. vitamin C for the gums:

Oranges, peppers and strawberries are rich in vitamin C, which plays a crucial role in gum health by supporting its strength and elasticity.

4. vitamin D - The sunshine vitamin:

Salmon, egg yolks and fortified dairy products are great sources of vitamin D, which improves the body's ability to absorb calcium, an essential building block for tooth enamel.

5. tea as a natural enemy of bacteria:

Black and green tea contain polyphenols that can inhibit the growth of bacteria that cause tooth decay and gum disease.

6. beware of sugary and acidic foods:

Sugar is the main food for harmful oral bacteria that produce acids and attack tooth enamel. Soft drinks, juices and even some sports drinks can have similar harmful effects.

7. whole grain products for a healthy mouth:

Whole grain products such as oatmeal, brown rice and whole wheat bread are rich in vitamin B and iron, which contribute to gum health.

8. moderation with alcohol and coffee:

Excessive alcohol and coffee consumption can lead to drying of the mouth, increasing the risk of tooth decay and other oral diseases.

9. fluoridated water:

Drinking fluoridated water can help strengthen tooth enamel and prevent tooth decay.

Conclusion:

A balanced diet rich in vitamins, minerals and fresh foods does wonders for our oral health. Through conscious eating habits, we can not only make our smile shine, but also lay the foundation for lifelong oral health.

How to treat bad breath naturally

Bad breath, known medically as halitosis, is more than just an annoying problem. For many people, it can be a sign of more serious health problems and can also affect social and professional relationships. Fortunately, there are a variety of natural ways to combat this unpleasant problem. Let's take a look at some of them:

1. good oral hygiene:

Let's start with the obvious. Brushing your teeth twice a day, in the morning and evening, and flossing are basic requirements. Particular attention should be paid to the tongue, as this is where many bacteria settle that can cause bad breath.

2. drink, drink, drink:

Adequate hydration helps keep the mouth moist and reduce bad odors. Water rinses food residues and bacteria out of the mouth that could otherwise lead to bad breath.

3. chew herbs:

Parsley, basil, mint and coriander contain chlorophyll, which acts as a natural deodorant. A small bunch after a meal can work wonders.

4th apple a day:

Chewing crunchy fruits or vegetables such as apples, carrots or celery can help remove plaque from teeth and stimulate saliva flow, which fights bad breath.

5. natural mouthwashes:

A mouthwash made of water and a few drops of tea tree oil or peppermint oil can work wonders. Rinsing with green tea, which has antibacterial properties, can also be effective.

6. probiotic foods:

Yogurt and other fermented foods can help reduce the growth of bad bacteria in the mouth. Look for products without added sugar.

7. avoid tobacco:

In addition to the many health hazards associated with smoking, tobacco is also a major cause of bad breath.

8. be careful with sugary drinks and alcohol:

Sugar provides a food source for bad bacteria in the mouth, while alcohol can dry out the mouth - both are major causes of bad breath.

Now let's turn to other practical and natural ways you can keep your breath fresh.

1. oil pulling:

This age-old Ayurvedic technique involves rinsing the mouth with a tablespoon of coconut or sesame oil for about 15-20 minutes and then spitting the oil out. It is said to draw bacteria and toxins out of the mouth. Be careful not to swallow the oil and then rinse the mouth well with water.

2. sodium bicarbonate:

A teaspoon of baking soda dissolved in a glass of water can serve as a mouthwash. Soda neutralizes acids and fights bacteria in the mouth. It can also be sprinkled on the toothbrush and used for brushing teeth.

3. abstaining from certain foods:

Some foods, such as onions and garlic, are known to cause bad breath. They can enter the lungs through the bloodstream and emit an unpleasant odor when exhaled. Reduce your consumption of these foods if you know you will be in company in the near future.

4. activated carbon:

Activated charcoal has adsorbent properties, which means it can bind odors and bacteria to itself. There are toothpastes with activated charcoal that can help reduce bad breath.

5. herbal teas:

Teas like chamomile and fennel can not only have a calming effect, but also promote oral health and fight bad breath.

6. aloe vera gel:

Aloe vera has antimicrobial properties. A homemade mouthwash made of water, a few drops of aloe vera gel and peppermint oil can freshen breath.

7. sea salt rinse:

Gargling with a solution of warm water and sea salt can help kill harmful bacteria in the mouth and throat.

8. hydration:

Dry mouth can lead to bad breath. In addition to drinking water, sugar-free candies or chewing gum can help stimulate saliva production and keep the mouth moist.

Closing Thoughts:

Bad breath can be embarrassing for individuals, but in many cases it is easily treatable. With a combination of good oral hygiene and some of the natural methods presented here, you can be assured of fresh breath and the self-confidence that comes with a healthy smile.

The importance of early detection and prevention of oral diseases

Amidst the hustle and bustle of our daily lives, it can be easy to overlook the importance of regular dental visits and checkups. But the health of our mouths, and specifically the early detection of oral disease, should never be taken lightly. Why? Let's take a deep look.

1. provide for the future instead of after the fact:

Most oral diseases, if detected at an early stage, are much easier and less expensive to treat. In addition, early intervention can often prevent serious complications.

2. symptoms are deceptive:

Some oral diseases, such as the onset of tooth decay or gum disease, can be asymptomatic. This means you may already be developing disease without even realizing it.

3. health of the whole body:

Our oral health often reflects the overall health of the body. Diseases such as diabetes or heart disease may be associated with oral problems. So early detection of oral problems can also provide clues to other health problems.

4. prevention protects against pain:

Tooth or gum pain can be extremely unpleasant. Early detection and prevention can save you from such pain and the associated discomfort.

5. a smile speaks volumes:

A healthy smile is not only aesthetically pleasing, but also a sign of good general well-being. Early detection and prevention can help preserve that smile.

6. reduction of the risk of tooth loss:

Early detection of diseases such as periodontitis can help prevent tooth loss by intervening in time.

Closing Thoughts:

The old saying "prevention is better than cure" also applies to our oral health. Regular dental checkups, good daily oral care and awareness of the first signs of problems are crucial to maintaining the health and beauty of our smile for years to come. It's not just about looks, it's about deep health care that can save us from many future problems.

7. FAQs and myths about natural dental care

Our teeth are often at the center of our self-confidence. A bright smile opens doors, while dental pain and problems can significantly affect our daily lives. Natural dental care is becoming increasingly important as many people seek alternatives to traditional dental care. However, with this rise in interest comes numerous questions and misconceptions. Here are some of the most discussed topics:

1. can I brush my teeth with water only?

A common misconception is that clear water alone is enough to keep our teeth clean. Although water helps remove food debris and some bacteria, it alone is not enough to effectively fight plaque or bacteria that cause cavities. Natural toothpastes or powders can be a better alternative here.

2. are fluoride toothpastes harmful?

Fluoride is a frequently discussed topic. It has been proven to have caries-inhibiting properties. However, too much fluoride can lead to fluorosis (white spots on the teeth). A middle ground can be the use of a fluoride-free toothpaste and occasional professional fluoride treatments.

3. can oil pulling and mouth rinses replace my visit to the dentist?

Oil pulling, a practice that involves swishing an oil (usually coconut oil) back and forth in the mouth, has many adherents. It can help reduce bacteria and cleanse the mouth, but it in no way replaces a visit to the dentist or daily tooth brushing. Mouthwashes are similar.

4. is whitening my teeth with activated charcoal safe?

Activated charcoal is found in many natural teeth whitening products. It can remove surface stains, but if used too frequently, it can wear away tooth enamel. Moderate use is recommended.

5. are all natural toothpastes the same?

No, they vary in their ingredients and effectiveness. Some contain baking soda for gentle exfoliation, others essential oils for flavor and antibacterial action. It's important to check the ingredients and choose a toothpaste that fits your needs.

6. is dental floss really necessary?

Despite the growing popularity of interdental brushes and other cleaning tools, dental floss remains an indispensable tool in oral care. It reaches places that are often missed by brushes. For those looking for a natural alternative, floss is available made of silk or coated with vegetable waxes.

7. Can I chew gum to clean my teeth?

Chewing gum can stimulate saliva production, which in turn can help remove food debris and balance the pH in the mouth. But it's not a substitute for brushing your teeth. If you choose to chew gum, choose sugar-free varieties or those with xylitol, which has caries-inhibiting properties.

8. what is the effect of essential oils in dental care?

Some essential oils, such as tea tree oil or peppermint oil, have antibacterial properties. When used in rinses or toothpastes, they can help fight bacteria and provide fresh breath. But be careful: too much or improper use can cause irritation.

9. Can I make my own natural dental care products?

Yes, many people make their own toothpastes and rinses. It is important to be aware of the best ingredients and their proper amounts. Homemade products should also be made in small quantities and prepared fresh on a regular basis.

10. do I need fewer dental visits with natural dental care?

A regular visit to the dentist is essential, regardless of the type of dental care you practice. A dentist can detect early signs of problems and recommend appropriate treatments.

Concluding considerations of this section:

Making an informed decision about dental care requires both knowledge and an understanding of your own needs. Nature offers many wonderful tools and resources to care for our teeth. But it is important to use them wisely and in combination with modern dental practices. Always remember that prevention is the key to a long and healthy smile.

Scientific findings and evidence for natural dental care

Modern dentistry has made impressive progress in recent decades, but more and more people are turning to natural dental care methods. But what does science say about such practices?

1. green tea and gum health

Green tea has been known for its health-promoting properties for centuries. Studies have shown that the catechins contained in green tea can protect the gums from inflammation and protect the mouth from harmful bacteria.

2. xylitol against caries

Xylitol, a natural sugar substitute, has been shown in studies to be effective against caries bacteria. Regular consumption can help reduce acidity in the mouth and thus minimize the risk of caries.

3. sage and oral health

Traditionally, sage was used for gargling or as an infusion to cleanse the mouth. Today, studies confirm the antimicrobial properties of sage, which can help inhibit the growth of harmful bacteria in the mouth.

4. oil pulling - More than just a trend?

Oil pulling, a traditional method from Ayurvedic medicine, has gained popularity in recent years. It involves swishing oil back and forth in the mouth to remove toxins. Although scientific results are mixed, many people report whiter teeth and healthier gums after regular practice.

5. coconut oil against bacteria

Coconut oil contains lauric acid, which has shown antibacterial properties in studies. This can help prevent the growth of harmful bacteria in the mouth.

6. neem - a traditional miracle cure

The neem tree is highly valued in traditional Indian medicine. Scientific studies support its use in inhibiting plaque formation and bacterial growth in the mouth.

7. activated carbon for white teeth?

Activated charcoal has gained popularity in natural dental care, especially for whitening teeth. Although some users report positive results, scientists emphasize the need for further research on the long-term effects on tooth enamel.

Final thoughts:

The world of natural dental care is rich with possibilities and discoveries. While many traditional methods are now validated by science, it is important to critically examine claims and combine the best of both worlds - traditional and modern. It is always advisable to consult a dental professional before making any major changes to your dental care routine.

Myths and facts about natural dental care

In the world of dental care, there are numerous stories and recommendations that have been passed down from generation to generation. But what is truth and what is fairy tale? Let's dive into some common myths and uncover the scientific facts behind them.

Myth 1: Lemon juice naturally whitens teeth.

Fact: Lemon juice contains citric acid, which can erode tooth enamel. Long-term use can lead to tooth sensitivity and is not recommended.

Myth 2: Baking soda is a safe and natural substitute for toothpaste.

Fact: While baking soda can effectively remove stains, its abrasive nature is potentially harmful to tooth enamel when used frequently. It should be used with caution and not as a regular alternative to toothpaste.

Myth 3: Oil pulling replaces tooth brushing.

Fact: Oil pulling can reduce bacteria and freshen the mouth, but should not replace daily brushing with fluoride toothpaste.

Myth 4: Aloe vera gel can cure gum disease.

Fact: Aloe vera has anti-inflammatory properties and can help with gingivitis, but "cure" is a strong word. It should be

considered as a supplement and not a substitute for professional treatment.

Myth 5: Sugar-free chewing gums are just a marketing gimmick
and offer no benefits for the teeth.

Fact: Sugar-free chewing gums, especially those with xylitol, can
actually help neutralize the pH in the mouth and prevent tooth
decay.

Myth 6: Herbal tinctures are just as effective as mouthwashes
from the pharmacy.

Fact: While some herbal tinctures have antimicrobial properties,
their effectiveness varies. Not all are as effective as commercial
mouthwashes.

Myth 7: A branch of a neem tree is a sufficient toothbrush substitute.

Fact: In many cultures, a neem sprig is traditionally used to
clean teeth. It has antimicrobial properties, but mechanical removal of plaque by modern toothbrushes is superior.

Conclusion:

With all the information that reaches us every day, it is important
to distinguish myths from facts. Natural dental care can be

effective, but it is essential to be well informed and to consult a dental professional if you are unsure.

How to switch from conventional to natural dental care

The journey from conventional to natural dental care can be an exciting one. It opens the doors to a world centered on the forces of nature and traditional wisdom. Before jumping in at the deep end, however, there are some steps and considerations that can help make the transition smooth and effective.

1. get informed:

Before making any change, it is important to do sound research. Read books, articles and studies that deal with natural dental care. It is critical to distinguish between well-researched sources and those that may not offer the best advice.

2. evaluation of the current products:

Take a close look at what products you are currently using. Some conventional products may already contain natural ingredients, while others are filled with chemicals you may want to avoid. Make a list and decide which products you want to replace first.

3. step by step change:

Abrupt change can be overwhelming and is not always the best approach. Start by replacing one product at a time with a natural alternative. That way, you can evaluate the effect of each new product on your oral health individually.

4. introduction of natural ingredients:

There are many natural ingredients that can be beneficial for oral health. Coconut oil, aloe vera, green tea and sage are just a few examples. Find out how to incorporate these into your daily dental care routine.

5. DIY - Self is the man:

One of the joys of natural dental care is the ability to make your own products. From toothpastes to mouthwashes, there are numerous recipes that are easy to try and effective.

Now that you're familiar with the basics of natural dental care, we'll dive deeper into some of the more specific aspects and practices. This will help you get a comprehensive overview of what it really means to switch to natural dental care.

1. natural tooth cleaning alternatives:

a. Miswak sticks: A traditional cleaning tool made from the Salvadora persica tree, used in many cultures for centuries. The stick is moistened and used like a toothbrush.

b. Oil pulling: This ancient Ayurvedic method involves rinsing the mouth with coconut or sesame oil for 10-20 minutes in the morning.

2. fluoride-free toothpaste:

There are concerns about the long-term use of fluoride. Many natural toothpastes instead rely on ingredients such as baking soda, salt or activated charcoal to gently clean and whiten teeth.

3. natural mouthwashes:

A mixture of water, essential oils (e.g. peppermint or tea tree) and salt can serve as an effective natural mouthwash. It can fight bacteria and freshen breath without disturbing the oral flora.

4. copper or stainless steel tongue scraper:

Tongue cleaning is an important step that is often overlooked. A tongue scraper can help effectively remove bacteria and debris that cause bad breath.

5. change of diet:

Diet plays a crucial role in dental health. Eating foods low in sugar and rich in nutrients, especially those rich in calcium and vitamin D, can significantly promote dental health.

6. continuous education:

Natural dental care is constantly evolving. New research and discoveries can offer helpful insights. It is therefore important to always stay up-to-date and be open to new techniques and information.

Making the switch from conventional to natural dental care is not just a simple product swap. It requires a holistic view of oral hygiene, nutrition and homemade preparations. It is a commitment to health and well-being that is rewarded with the right guidance and the will to change.

Final thoughts

Summary of the main points and principles of natural dental care.

1. holistic approach:

Natural dental care considers not only the teeth in isolation, but the whole body. It is about creating a harmonious balance between oral flora, nutrition and overall health.

2. minimization of chemical influences:

Instead of aggressive, synthetic substances, natural dental care products rely on ingredients from nature that clean gently and effectively.

3. prevention instead of reaction:

While conventional approaches often aim to treat problems after they have occurred, natural dental care focuses on preventing potential discomfort in the first place.

4. nutrition as the key:

A low-sugar, mineral- and vitamin-rich diet protects teeth and promotes healthy gums. A balanced diet can significantly reduce tooth decay and gum problems.

5. return to traditional methods:

Old techniques such as oil pulling or the use of miswak sticks are being rediscovered and integrated into modern natural dental care as effective means.

6. respect for the oral flora:

Instead of aggressively fighting bacteria in the mouth, a harmonious environment is created where beneficial bacteria thrive and harmful bacteria are naturally regulated.

7. environmental awareness:

Many natural dental care products rely on environmentally friendly packaging and sustainable ingredients. This not only protects your own body, but also our planet.

8. continuous learning:

Natural dental care is not a rigid concept. It is constantly evolving, and followers are often keen to stay on top of the latest research.

In conclusion, natural dental care is much more than just an alternative to conventional care. It is a philosophy that focuses on health, sustainability and respect for one's own body and the environment. With the principles presented here, everyone has the opportunity to find their way to healthier and more conscious dental care.

Afterword

Dear Readers,

together we have taken a journey through the depths and possibilities of natural dental care. You may now be asking yourself how you can integrate the knowledge gained into your life in the long term. It is one thing to learn something new, but another to implement it consistently and permanently.

The key is motivation. Why did you choose this book? Perhaps you are looking for gentler alternatives to conventional dental care, perhaps you are striving for a more conscious and nature-loving lifestyle, or perhaps, like me, you have had your own experiences with intolerances. Always keep your personal reasons in mind. Every time you reach for your new, natural toothpaste or use one of the methods presented, remind yourself why you chose this path.

But motivation alone is not always enough. To permanently integrate natural dental care into your everyday life, you also need a routine. Start gradually. Don't change everything at once, but add a new habit every week. Maybe start by replacing conventional toothpaste with a natural alternative. Then the following week you could introduce an oil pulling regimen, and so on.

Talk to others about your experiences and exchange ideas. Share your experiences of success and also your challenges. A community, even if only in a small circle, can work wonders to keep you going.

Finally, I would like to give you the following advice: Be patient with yourself. Every change takes time. There will be days when you doubt and others when you will clearly feel the positive effects. But no matter what obstacles you face, always remember that you have chosen a path that benefits not only your mouth, but your entire body and our environment.

Thank you from the bottom of my heart for your trust and guidance on this path. May natural dental care become more than just a method for you - may it become an integral and enriching part of your lifestyle.

With warm regards and best wishes for your health,

Jessica F. Turner.